THE LATEST GLOBAL HEALTH THREAT– NEUROLOGICAL DISORDERS:

A comprehensive health awareness guide on neurological disorders that reveals the symptoms, causes, and treatments of over

30 neurological illnesses.

By

Dr. Robert J. Cardwell

All rights reserved. Copyright © by Dr. Robert J. Cardwell 2024.

Except for brief quotations included in critical reviews and specific noncommercial uses allowed by copyright law, no part of this book may be duplicated, distributed, or transmitted in any way or by any means, including photocopying, recording, or other electronic or mechanical methods, without the author's prior written permission.

Table of Contents

THE LATEST GLOBAL HEALTH THREAT– NEUROLOGICAL DISORDERS: 1

All rights reserved. Copyright © by Dr. Robert J. Cardwell 2024. 2

Introduction. 6

Chapter 1 15

Pathology of Neurological Disorders. 15

Chapter 2 22

Concept and Instructions of WHO on Neurological Disorders. 22

   The effect of neurological disorders globally 24

Chapter 3 28

Neurological disorders; symptoms, causes, and treatments. 28

   Alzheimer's disease 28

    Stroke 38

Chapter 4 42

Traumatic Brain Injury (TBI) 42

   Symptoms 43

Chapter 5	**52**
Muscular Dystrophy	**54**
Chapter 6	**63**
Restless Legs Syndrome	**63**
Peripheral Neuropathy	**65**
Facial Nerve Palsy (Bell's palsy)	**67**
Chapter 7	**72**
Autoimmune Encephalitis	**72**
Chapter 8	**81**
Spinocerebellar Ataxia.	**81**
Autism Spectrum Disorder (ASD).	**85**
Chapter 9	**90**
Meningitis	**90**
Dementia	**92**
ND(s) Associated with Preterm Birth.	**94**
Chapter 10	**100**
Four Major Brain Disorders Concerning Neurological Disorders	**100**
How New Neurological Disorder and FRYL Gene Variant are associated.	**102**

Neurocrine Bioscience Therapy 107
Conclusion 110

Introduction

A class of illnesses known as neurological disorders impacts the brain, spinal cord, and nerves throughout the body. These illnesses may present in many ways, from minor symptoms to incapacitating problems that significantly impair a person's quality of life. Given that millions of individuals worldwide suffer from neurological issues, it is critical to comprehend the conditions' origins, signs, and potential therapies.

This introduction will examine the incidence of neurological illnesses in American society and how they affect people and their families. We will also investigate the prevalence of neurological diseases worldwide and the initiatives to address this expanding public health concern.

Neurological Disorders in America

The Latest Global Health Threat – Neurological Disorders

Each year, millions of Americans suffer from neurological illnesses; among the most prevalent are multiple sclerosis, epilepsy, Alzheimer's disease, Parkinson's disease, and Parkinson's disease. Nearly one in six Americans, according to the National Institute of Neurological Disorders and Stroke, suffer from a neurological illness. As the population ages, this figure is projected to rise.

According to significant new research published in The Lancet Neurology, over 3 billion individuals globally had a neurological illness in 2021. The World Health Organization (WHO) contributed to analyzing the Global Burden of Disease, Injuries, and Risk Factor Study.

In the world today, neurological illnesses are the primary cause of disability and the second most significant cause of mortality. According to a ground-breaking new Global Burden of Illness (GBD) research, by 2050, there will be twice as many individuals with brain illness.

"The research indicates that more than 40% of people worldwide presently experience a neurological disorder, and this number is expected to almost quadruple by 2050," says Dr. Valery Feigin, an epidemiologist and neurology professor at the National Institute for Stroke and Applied Neurosciences at Auckland University of Technology. "This is a warning: the entire health system will collapse if we do not take adequate action to combat neurological disorders."

Feigin presented the results of the Global Burden of Disease (GBD) study. The goal of the GBD research is to assist inform healthcare and policy choices at national and international levels. It is the most thorough attempt to date to map the worldwide burden of neurological illnesses.

The Top 10 Most Disabling Neurological Conditions in the World, According to the GBD Study

The GBD study offers estimates on the prevalence, years lived with disability (YLDs), years of life lost (YLLs), and disability-adjusted life-years (DALYs) for each of the 36 most prevalent neurological illnesses and conditions in the world.

Currently, 90% of all neurological DALYs are caused by ten conditions:

Stroke

Neonatal encephalopathy

Migraine

Dementia

Meningitis

Epilepsy

Neurological complications associated with preterm birth

Nervous system cancers (brain tumors).

Autism spectrum disorders

Parkinson's disease

According to Feigin, "these illnesses were the top ten global contributors to nervous system burden." "We can significantly lower the worldwide burden if we concentrate on treating these ten illnesses, but study is still needed to determine the causes, risk factors, best therapies, and rehabilitation techniques."

Globally and nationally, healthcare strategies, policies, financing, and training will be influenced by the GBD research. Additionally, it will advance knowledge of the global impact of neurological illnesses.

Neurological illnesses may significantly affect patients and their families; symptoms can include mobility and motor function loss, cognitive decline, and memory loss. These symptoms may dramatically impair an individual's capacity to carry out everyday tasks, engage in employment, and engage in social relationships, resulting in depressive and isolated sentiments.

A considerable financial burden is also attributed to neurological illnesses in addition to their cost. Care for people with neurological problems may be expensive; prescription drugs, medical appointments, and specialist equipment can rapidly mount up in costs. It is estimated that the annual cost of care for those with neurological illnesses in the US is in the billions of dollars.

The Effects of Neurological Disorders globally

Neurological illnesses are a worldwide public health concern that impacts people in all nations, not just those in the United States. Neurological illnesses rank second globally in terms of the cause of mortality and the primary cause of disability, according to the World Health Organization. The enormous worldwide burden of neurological disorders is attributed to the estimated one billion individuals who live with these ailments.

The effect of neurological illnesses might be even more severe in low- and middle-income nations because of the lack of access to resources and healthcare facilities. Delays in diagnosis and treatment may result from this, and people with neurological illnesses may face more stigma and prejudice as a result. Many individuals in these nations may not get the assistance and treatment necessary to manage their conditions as a consequence properly.

Despite these obstacles, the significance of

treating neurological illnesses globally is becoming more apparent. Organizations like the World Health Organization and the Global Burden of Disease Study have been striving to increase public awareness of these problems and encourage research and cooperation to improve treatment and outcomes for people with neurological illnesses.

Neurological illnesses have an immense effect on individuals, families, and communities and are a significant public health concern that affects millions of people in the US and throughout the globe. Improving the quality of life for people with neurological illnesses requires understanding the problems' origins, symptoms, and accessible therapies.

In the following sections, we will detail certain neurological conditions, including their causes, symptoms, and available treatments. We will also discuss the most recent findings and developments in neurology and the difficulties and chances associated with reducing the prevalence of neurological illnesses worldwide. By banding together to spread knowledge, encourage research, and foster cooperation, we can improve the lives of those who suffer from neurological diseases.

Would you want to know more about neurological conditions and how people are affected globally? For a thorough examination of the origins, signs, and treatments of neurological diseases and the effects these problems have on people and their families, turn no further than the comprehensive awareness book "The Global Health Threat". By reading this book, you will acquire ideal knowledge of the intricacies of neurological illnesses and improve your understanding of how to manage and treat these problems.

Furthermore, I am grateful for your enthusiasm for reading The Recent Global Threat to Health—Neurological Disorders. I hope you find my work exciting and educational. Your interest in it means a lot to me.

Comments from readers such as yourselves are helpful to me as an author. I would appreciate it if you could read the book and write a review to share your opinions. Your review may help others find the book and provide me with insightful information for my following writing projects.

Chapter 1
Pathology of Neurological Disorders.

A broad spectrum of illnesses that impact the brain, spinal cord, and nerves and cause abnormalities in normal neurological function are referred to as neurological diseases. To effectively manage these complicated illnesses, it is essential to comprehend the pathophysiology of neurological disorders and create therapies and interventions accordingly. In this scientific explanation, we shall examine neurological illnesses' clinical characteristics and underlying mechanisms, emphasizing important facets of cellular pathology, neuroanatomy, and molecular processes related to these problems.

Neuroanatomy and Cellular Pathology.

The human nervous system is an intricate web of linked cells and structures that controls many vital bodily processes. The brain, which comprises the brainstem, cerebellum, and cerebrum, is essential for coordinating motor, memory, sensory perception, and cognitive functions. The spinal cord facilitates movement, sensation, and reflexes as a channel for messages to be sent from the brain to the body's other organs. From the spinal cord, nerves innervate muscles and organs, facilitating appropriate bodily function and coordination.

Deviations from these brain components' standard structure or function might result in neurological diseases. For instance, the gradual loss of neurons and synapses in specific brain areas characterizes neurodegenerative illnesses like Alzheimer's and Parkinson's, which results in cognitive decline and movement difficulties. Myelin, the coating that protects nerve fibers, is destroyed by the immune system in inflammatory diseases such as multiple sclerosis, which causes abnormal signal transmission and neurological impairments. Pathology in neurological illnesses often entails changes in the structure and function of neurons at the cellular level. The main functional components of the nervous system, neurons, use complex signaling mechanisms to send and receive information electrochemically.

Neurological dysfunction may result from aberrant neurotransmitter release or poor synaptic connection, which are examples of disruptions in neuronal signaling pathways that affect neural transmission. Furthermore, glial cells are essential for preserving the neuronal environment and reacting to damage or illness because they shield and support neurons.

Molecular Processes and Pathophysiology:

Neurological illnesses are caused by complex molecular mechanisms involving complex cellular processes that control signaling pathways, protein synthesis, and gene expression. By upsetting the delicate balance of molecular interactions within the nervous system, genetic mutations, environmental influences, and epigenetic modifications may contribute to developing neurological illnesses.
Aberrant protein aggregation and misfolding are essential aspects of the pathophysiology of neurodegenerative disorders. For example, the build-up of tau tangles and amyloid-beta plaques

in the brain causes neuroinflammation and interferes with regular neuronal activity in Alzheimer's disease. Analogously, oxidative stress, mitochondrial malfunction, and neuronal death result from the aggregation of alpha-synuclein protein in dopaminergic neurons in Parkinson's disease.

Inflammatory processes also play a role in the pathophysiology of neurological illnesses by inducing immune responses that harm brain tissues. In multiple sclerosis, immune cells invade the central nervous system and target myelin, causing demyelination and axonal degeneration. Producing pro-inflammatory cytokines and chemokines in chronic inflammatory situations intensifies neuroinflammation and prolongs neuronal damage.

Future Paths and Therapeutic Strategies.
Comprehending the pathophysiology of neurological illnesses is essential to creating focused treatment plans that target these ailments' underlying molecular and cellular processes.

Current therapy options include neuroprotection, disease modification, and symptom management to reduce symptoms and delay the course of neurological illnesses. The goal of pharmacological treatments, such as immunomodulatory medicines for multiple sclerosis or dopaminergic pharmaceuticals for Parkinson's disease, is to modify specific pathways linked to the pathophysiology of the illness.

Novel therapeutic modalities such as stem cell transplantation, gene therapy, and precision medicine provide encouraging prospects for tailored management of neurological conditions. CRISPR-Cas9 and other gene editing technologies have the potential to repair genetic abnormalities linked to neurodegenerative illnesses and return neurons to their normal function. In diseases like spinal cord injury or stroke, stem cell-based treatments provide the chance to replace lost or malfunctioning cells and regenerate damaged brain structures.

The origin and evolution of neurological illnesses are thus attributed to the intricate interaction of neuroanatomical, cellular, and molecular mechanisms that make up their pathology. Technological and scientific developments reveal the complex processes behind neurological illness, opening the door to novel treatment modalities and individualized therapies. By clarifying the pathological underpinnings of neurological disorders, clinicians and researchers may better understand disease processes, increase diagnosis accuracy, and improve treatment results for persons afflicted by these problematic illnesses.

The field of medicine known as neurology is concerned with diagnosing, evaluating, and managing conditions of the nervous system, which comprises the brain, spinal cord, and nerves. Neurology involves the diagnosis and treatment of many problems of the nervous system, including headaches, epilepsy, strokes, neurodegenerative diseases, and abnormalities of the peripheral nerves.

Understanding the intricate functions of the brain and nervous system requires a multidisciplinary approach in neurology. Information from many disciplines, including neuroanatomy, neurophysiology, neurochemistry, and neuroimaging, is integrated. Neurologists are medical professionals who specialize in diagnosing and treating neurological problems. They do this by using a variety of diagnostic tests, physical examinations, and medical histories to diagnose patients and provide individualized treatment programs accurately.

To sum up, neurology is a branch of science that studies the nervous system and the brain. The ultimate objective is to treat and understand neurological problems to maximize a person's health and well-being.

Chapter 2
Concept and Instructions of WHO on Neurological Disorders.

Neurological diseases are recognized by the World Health Organization (WHO) as a significant global health burden that impacts millions of people globally. Based on WHO estimates, neurological illnesses represent a substantial share of the world's disease burden, with prevalence rates differing across people and geographical areas. The WHO's viewpoint on neurological illnesses and the present numbers of Americans and other people worldwide who suffer from them is summarized as follows:

Worldwide Burden.
Diseases related to the nervous system, such as epilepsy, stroke, Alzheimer's, and Parkinson's, account for a large portion of the world's illness and disability burden.
- Neurological illnesses are the second most significant cause of mortality globally and the leading cause of disability, according to statistics from the World Health Organization.

It is anticipated that as the population ages and the frequency of non-communicable illnesses rises, the prevalence of neurological disorders will increase as well, putting an increasing strain on healthcare systems and society.

Statistics of Neurological Disorders in America
- Neurological problems afflict millions of people in the United States, affecting people of all ages with various ailments.
- The Centers for Disease Control and Prevention (CDC) estimate that 1 in 6 adult Americans suffers from a neurological ailment; frequent disorders include dementia, epilepsy, and migraines.
- In America, neurological illnesses are linked to high healthcare expenditures, disability, and a lower standard of living for those who are afflicted and their family.

The effect of neurological disorders globally
Millions of individuals worldwide are thought to be affected by neurological illnesses, with prevalence rates differing across locations and nations.

- Neurological illnesses are more common in low- and middle-income nations, where there is less access to resources, healthcare, and specialist services for diagnosis and treatment.
- The WHO underlines the need for improved awareness, research, and investment in these conditions to address the increasing global health concerns of neurological illnesses.

The World Health Organization concludes by stressing the severe effects of neurological diseases on health worldwide and the need for all-encompassing approaches to the care, diagnosis, and prevention of these challenging illnesses. By boosting research, bolstering healthcare systems, and increasing public awareness of these disorders, the World Health Organization seeks to lessen the worldwide burden of neurological diseases and improve outcomes for those impacted.

Here is a thorough list of the most common neurological conditions:

1. Alzheimer's Disease
2. Parkinson's Disease
3. Epilepsy
4. Multiple Sclerosis
5. Stroke
6. Migraines
7. Traumatic Brain Injury
8. Huntington's Disease
9. Amyotrophic Lateral Sclerosis (ALS)
10. Cerebral Palsy
11. Neurodegenerative Diseases (e.g. ALS, Parkinson's, Alzheimer's)
12. Brain Tumors
13. Muscular Dystrophy
14. Spinal Muscular Atrophy

15. Myasthenia Gravis

16. Tourette syndrome

17. Restless Legs Syndrome

18. Peripheral Neuropathy

19. Bell's Palsy

20. Transverse Myelitis

21. Autoimmune Encephalitis

22. Creutzfeldt-Jakob Disease

23. Neurofibromatosis

24. Rett Syndrome

25. Spinocerebellar Ataxia

26. Friedreich's Ataxia

27. Autism spectrum disorders

28. Meningitis

29. Dementia

30. Neurological complications associated with preterm birth.

31. Neonatal encephalopathy.

While many additional neurological illnesses exist, this list highlights some of the most common ones. Notably, every condition might exhibit diverse symptoms and intensities, necessitating a tailored medical assessment and course of action.

Chapter 3

Neurological disorders; symptoms, causes, and treatments.

Alzheimer's disease

Alzheimer's is a degenerative neurological condition that impairs thinking, behavior, and memory. It is the most typical cause of dementia, a collection of illnesses that affect the brain and cause cognitive ability to decrease. The hallmark of Alzheimer's disease is the buildup of aberrant protein deposits in the brain, which cause nerve cell death and brain tissue degradation.

Symptoms:

Disruptive memory loss in day-to-day activities
- Having trouble doing routine chores
- Difficulties in organizing or solving problems
- Doubt about the date or location
- Modifications to personality or mood
- Losing the capacity to trace back steps and misplacing objects

Causes:

- The buildup of protein plaques and tangles in the brain, which cause nerve cell death and brain tissue loss, is the hallmark of Alzheimer's disease. Alzheimer's disease is partly hereditary, with some genes, including APOE-e4, increasing the risk.
- The majority of individuals with Alzheimer's disease are 65 years of age or older, making age a substantial risk factor.

Treatments:

- Alzheimer's disease cannot be cured, but symptoms may be managed, and the illness's course can be slowed.
- Drugs like cholinesterase inhibitors (like rivastigmine and donepezil) may help control symptoms and enhance cognitive performance.
- Lifestyle modifications, such as consistent exercise, a balanced diet, social interaction, and mental stimulation, may help enhance the quality of life for those suffering from Alzheimer's disease.
- Support for caregivers and behavioral therapy are also crucial components in managing Alzheimer's

Parkinson's disease

Parkinson's disease is a degenerative neurological condition marked by stiffness, tremors, and impaired movement and coordination.

Symptoms

- Tremors, which often begin in a hand or limb
- Bradykinesia, characterized by sluggishness
- Stiffness or rigidity in the trunk or limbs
- Decreased coordination and equilibrium
Modifications to writing and speaking

Causes:

- Although the precise etiology of Parkinson's disease is unclear, a mix of environmental and hereditary factors is thought to be involved.
One of the main features of Parkinson's disease is the loss of dopamine-producing neurons in the brain. Motor symptoms result from aberrant brain activity brought on by this dopamine depletion.

Treatments:

Medication: Dopamine replacement therapy is often used to treat symptoms. Different drugs may also alleviate tremors, stiffness, and other symptoms.

Deep Brain Stimulation: To assist in controlling aberrant brain activity, electrodes are surgically

inserted into the brain.
- Exercise and Physical Therapy: Regular exercise and physical therapy may enhance mobility, flexibility, and balance.
- Speech Therapy: Speech therapy is helpful for those with Parkinson's disease who have trouble swallowing and speaking.
Lifestyle Modifications: People with Parkinson's disease may also control their symptoms and live better by eating a balanced diet, exercising, and maintaining social ties.

Epilepsy

The neurological condition known as epilepsy is characterized by recurring seizures that are brought on by aberrant brain electrical activity.

Symptoms:

- Seizures: Recurrent seizures, which may vary in severity, length, and kind, are the defining sign of epilepsy. Seizures may manifest as convulsions, unconsciousness, or strange feelings.

- Momentary confusion: People may suffer from memory loss, disorientation, and momentary confusion after a seizure.
- Uncontrollably jerky arm and leg movements: A person experiencing a seizure may experience uncontrollably jerky arm or leg movements or other body parts.

Temporary loss of consciousness or awareness: A person experiencing a seizure may lose consciousness or awareness, impairing their capacity to engage with their surroundings.
- Psychic symptoms: Fear, déjà vu, or unexplainable feelings are examples of psychic symptoms that may accompany some kinds of - seizures. These are personal experiences that differ from person to person.
- Repetitive motions: Lip-smacking, eye blinking, and hand rubbing are examples of repetitive movements caused by some types of epilepsy.

Causes:

- Idiopathic: A lot of people with epilepsy have idiopathic epilepsy, which is categorized as

having no recognized etiology.
- Hereditary factors: Certain gene mutations may predispose people to seizure disorders, and in certain circumstances, there is a hereditary component to epilepsy.
- Brain traumas: Epilepsy may be brought on by infections, brain tumors, strokes, and traumatic brain injuries.
- Developmental disorders: Epilepsy risk may be elevated by conditions such as Down syndrome, cerebral palsy, and autism spectrum disorder.
- Illnesses: Many illnesses, including encephalitis and meningitis, may cause inflammation in the brain and consequent seizures.
- Birth trauma: Postpartum complications, such as brain oxygen starvation, may lead to epilepsy in later life.

Treatments:

- Anti-seizure drugs: Anti-seizure drugs help control or prevent seizures and are the mainstay of therapy for epilepsy.
- Surgery: To eliminate the area of the brain

causing seizures when drugs are not working, this option may be explored.
- Vagus nerve stimulation: This treatment may help lower the frequency of seizures by implanting a device that stimulates the vagus nerve with electrical impulses.
- Ketogenic diet: Research has shown that a high-fat, low-carb ketogenic diet is effective in lowering seizures in some epileptic patients.
- Lifestyle changes: Epilepsy may be managed by avoiding triggers, keeping a regular sleep pattern, controlling stress, and abstaining from alcohol and illegal substances.
- Alternative Treatments: To supplement conventional methods, some people look into alternative therapies like acupuncture, biofeedback, or relaxation techniques.

Due to the complexity of epilepsy, treatment regimens must be customized to the distinctive symptoms, underlying reasons, and medical background of each patient. To successfully manage epilepsy and enhance quality of life, regular monitoring and communication with healthcare specialists are crucial.

Multiple Sclerosis (MS).

Multiple sclerosis (MS) is a long-term neurological disorder that affects the central nervous system. The immune system erroneously attacks the protective coating of nerve fibers, resulting in various physical and cognitive problems.

Symptoms

- Exhaustion

- One or more limbs experiencing numbness or weakness

- Shaking or incoordination

- Feelings of electric shock while moving the neck - Speech slurred

 - Visual issues (double vision, fuzzy vision, loss of eyesight) Sensations of pain or tingling in different bodily areas

- Cognitive abnormalities (difficulties with memory, concentration, thinking, or problem-solving)

- Problems with bowel or bladder movements

- Sadness or fluctuations in mood

Causes

Although the precise etiology of multiple sclerosis is uncertain, it is thought to be an inflammatory illness in which the immune system destroys the coating that protects nerve fibers, known as the myelin sheath.

Treatments

Drugs to control symptoms and halt the disease's development

- Corticosteroids to lessen swelling when relapses occur - Treatments that change the disease to reduce the severity and frequency of relapses

- Physical treatment to enhance coordination, strength, and balance

- Occupational therapy to help with day-to-day functioning

- speaking therapy for issues with swallowing and speaking

- Counseling and psychotherapy to treat mental and emotional disorders.

Patients with multiple sclerosis must collaborate closely with their medical team to develop a customized treatment plan that addresses their unique symptoms and requirements.

Stroke

A stroke is an abrupt stoppage of blood flow to the brain, which may damage brain tissue and produce a range of neurological symptoms.

Symptoms:

- Abrupt weak point or numbness inside the wrist, leg, or face, regularly on one body aspect.

- Abrupt disorientation, difficulties speaking or comprehending speech.

- Abrupt imaginative and prescient loss in a single or each eye

- Abrupt trouble walking, lightheadedness, unsteadiness, or loss of coordination.

- An abrupt, intense headache without a recognized cause.

Causes

Ischemic Stroke: Resulting from a blood clot or other obstruction in a blood artery providing blood to the brain.

Hemorrhagic Stroke: A blood artery break that causes brain hemorrhage.

Transient Ischemic Attack (TIA): Often referred to as a "mini-stroke," TIAs are brought on by a transient blockage that eventually clears up.

Treatments

> Ischemic Cerebrovascular Accident:

- Drugs called thrombolytics that break up blood clots

- Methods of mechanical clot removal.

- Antiplatelet drugs to stop new clot formation

> Stroke with hemorrhage:

- Vascular surgery to repair broken blood vessels

- Coiling or cutting to stop more bleeding

- Controlling blood pressure to stop bleeding again.

> TIA:

- Reducing risk factors, including smoking, diabetes, and high blood pressure.

- Antiplatelet drugs to lower the risk of stroke.

- Modifications to lifestyle, such as food and exercise, can enhance general health and lower the risk of stroke.

Migraine

Recurrent moderate to severe headaches are the hallmark of a migraine, a neurological disorder that is also often accompanied by light or sound sensitivity, nausea, and vomiting.

Symptoms

- Severe headache that pulses or throbs, generally on one side of the head.

- Stooling and queasiness.

- Sound and light sensitivity.

- In some instances, aura (flashes of light, blind patches, tingling in the extremities).

- Disturbances in vision.

- Vertigo or dizziness.

- Exhaustion or an allergy to certain scents Causes: - Genetic susceptibility.

 - Families are often affected by migraines.

 - Triggers include stress, hormonal shifts, certain meals or drinks, altered sleep habits, and external circumstances.

- Modifications to serotonin levels in the brain may impact blood vessel function and pain perception.

Treatments

Depending on the intensity and regularity of the episodes, there are many ways to treat migraines:

- Over-the-counter analgesics (acetaminophen, ibuprofen).

- Prescription pharmaceuticals (ergots, anti-nausea meds, triptans).

- Preventive drugs to lessen the frequency and intensity of migraines

- Lifestyle adjustments, such as stress reduction, consistent sleep schedules, and food adjustments

- Alternative treatments (such as biofeedback, acupuncture, and relaxation methods) Steer clear of recognized triggers, such as certain meals, beverages, or surroundings.

Together with their medical professionals, migraine sufferers should create a customized treatment plan that will enhance their quality of life while successfully managing their symptoms.

Chapter 4

Traumatic Brain Injury (TBI)

A blow, jolt, or penetrating damage to the head that causes an abrupt injury to the brain and results in either temporary or permanent neurological disability is known as a traumatic brain injury (TBI).

Symptoms
- A continual headache or strain in the head
- Feeling unclear or unfocused
- Loss of memory or trouble focusing
- Variations in behavior or mood

The Latest Global Health Threat – Neurological Disorders

- Tiredness or somnolence
Vomiting or feeling queasy
- Modifications to the senses (loss of eyesight, ringing in the ears)
- Trouble falling asleep or staying up later than normal

Causes
- Falls
- Car crashes
- Assaults
- Injuries sustained playing sports
- Detonation charges or more battlefield wounds
- Injury caused by items penetrating the skull

Treatments
- Quick medical intervention to stop bleeding and stop further injury
- Keep being cautious for warning signs and signs of extended intracranial pressure.
- Drugs to treat conditions including pain, convulsions, or mental problems
- Rehabilitation to enhance mental, emotional,

and physical abilities
- Support and counseling to help the person and their family deal with the changes that follow a traumatic brain injury.

Huntington disease

A degenerative neurological condition that impairs physical, cognitive, and mental abilities, Huntington's disease causes involuntary motions, cognitive impairment, and behavioral abnormalities.

Symptoms:
- Uncontrollably jerking or twitching (chorea)
- Modifications to balance and coordination
- Cognitive decline, including issues with concentration and memory
- Variations in mood, agitation, melancholy, or worry
- Issues with swallowing and speaking
- Rigidity or stiffness of the muscles
- Deteriorated fine motor abilities

- Modifications in behavior, impulsivity

Causes
A mutation in the genome that impacts the HTT gene
- The defective gene is inherited from one afflicted parent
- Depletion of certain brain chemicals

Treatments
- Symptomatic treatment, including the use of drugs to reduce movement and psychological problems

- Occupational and physical therapy to preserve mobility and function
- Speech therapy to help with communication problems
- Genetic counseling for vulnerable people and their families
- Supportive treatment to meet the patient's evolving demands as the illness worsens.

Amyotrophic Lateral Sclerosis (ALS)

Lou Gehrig's disease, commonly known as amyotrophic lateral sclerosis (ALS), is a neurodegenerative condition that progressively damages brain and spinal cord nerve cells, resulting in muscular weakness, paralysis, and, finally, loss of motor function.

Symptoms
- Weakness or stiffness in the muscles, commonly starting in the limbs
- Spasm or twitching of the muscles
- Trouble speaking, swallowing, or breathing
- Quick onset of symptoms that result in paralysis
- Atrophy or withering of muscles
- Uncontrollably laughing or sobbing or exhibiting erratic emotions
- In some instances, cognitive alterations

Causes
- Mutations in the genes encoding superoxide dismutase 1 (SOD1) and C9orf72
- Triggers or environmental variables might be

involved.
- Cellular malfunction and abnormal protein aggregation

Treatments
- The FDA has authorized riluzole and edaravone as drugs to halt the course of illness.
- Physical treatment to preserve muscle autonomy and function
- Communication aids and speech therapy for swallowing and speech problems
- Support for breathing when the illness worsens
- Multidisciplinary assistance and care to control symptoms and enhance life quality.

Cerebral Palsy

A set of conditions known as cerebral palsy impacts motor abilities, muscle tone, and movement. These problems are usually brought on by harm to the developing brain before, during, or soon after birth.

Symptoms

- Slower than expected motor skill development
- Flappiness or rigidity of the muscles
- Weak balance and coordination
- Involuntary motions or tremors
- Difficulties with fine motor abilities, such as buttoning garments or writing
- Language and speech delays
- Issues with hearing or vision
- In some instances, intellectual deficiencies

Causes
- Abnormalities or brain damage that develops before, during, or soon after birth
- Pregnancy-related infections, such as CMV or rubella
- Asphyxia, or lack of oxygen to the brain during birth
- Mutations or genetic factors
- Low birth weight or premature delivery

Treatments
- Physical treatment to enhance coordination and muscular strength

- Occupational remedy to help with day-by-day residing tasks
- Speech treatment to enhance verbal abilities
- Drugs to control seizures or spasticity
- Orthopedic procedures, such as surgery or braces
- Assistive technology, such as communication aids or wheelchairs
- Assistance with education for kids with cerebral palsy.

Neurodegenerative diseases

A class of illnesses known as neurodegenerative diseases is defined by the gradual death of nerve cells in the brain or peripheral nervous system, resulting in a range of symptoms, including impaired mobility, diminished cognitive function, and loss of sensory perception.

Symptoms
- A steady decline in cognitive abilities

- Deficits in motor function include tremors, muscle rigidity, and balance issues.
- Modifications in behavior, mood swings, and personality.
- Disorientation and memory loss.
- Speech, language, and communication difficulties.
- Deteriorated decision-making and executive function
- Modifications to perception or feeling.
- Tiredness and sleep issues.
- Misfolded and accumulated proteins in the brain.
- Genetic alterations in specific genes, such as those seen in Alzheimer's or Huntington's diseases.
- Environmental elements, such as poisons or brain trauma.
- Oxidative stress and inflammation are factors in neuronal damage.
- Cellular function changes associated with aging.

Treatments

- Using medicine to treat symptoms and reduce the rate at which the illness progresses
- Exercise and physical treatment to preserve function and mobility
Rehabilitating cognitive function and memories
- Supportive care to meet patients' and carers' requirements
- Investigations into treatments for diseases or possible remedies
- Lifestyle changes that support general well-being and brain function, such as a balanced diet and frequent exercise.

Chapter 5
Brain Tumors

Brain tumors are abnormal cell growths inside the brain that, depending on their location and size, may cause various symptoms. They can be benign (non-cancerous) or malignant (cancerous) and possibly compromise normal brain function.

Symptoms
- Headaches that become worse when you get up or when you move positions
- Convulsions
- Stooling and queasiness
- Modifications to speech, hearing, or vision
- Cognitive alterations, such as disorientation or memory loss
- A weakening or numbing of the extremities
- Shifts in personality or mood
- Issues with coordination and balance

Causes:
- Genetic susceptibility
- Being uncovered to ensure chemical compounds or radiation.
- Infections or illnesses of the immune system
- Environmental elements
- Brain tumors in the family history
- Gender and age (brain tumors are more common in males)

Treatments

- Surgery to cut off the growth
- Radiation treatment
- Chemotherapy
- Modified medication regimen
- Radiosurgery using stereotaxy
- Supportive treatment for adverse effects and symptoms
- Clinical studies for new therapeutic approaches.

Muscular Dystrophy

Muscular dystrophy is a class of hereditary diseases characterized by gradually weakening and degrading muscles. Over time, it causes the skeletal muscles to weaken, which causes disability.

Symptoms
- Progressive atrophy and weakening of the muscles
- Having trouble standing or walking
- Joint contractures and stiffness of the muscles
- Weak balance and coordination
- Spastic and cramping muscles

- Issues with breathing
- Heart issues
- A sluggish decline in ability over time

Causes
- Mutations in the DNA that impact proteins necessary for muscular contraction
- Genetic defects inherited from parents
- Dystrophin gene mutations causing Becker and Duchenne muscular dystrophy
- Additional genes related to the composition and operation of muscles in different forms of muscular dystrophy

Treatments:
- Physical treatment to keep muscles flexible and strong
- Occupational therapy to enhance abilities for everyday life
- Assistive equipment such as wheelchairs or braces
- Support for breathing when required
- Drugs to control symptoms and halt the spread

of the illness
- Clinical studies for gene therapy and other experimental therapies
- Multidisciplinary team management and supportive care to provide the best possible quality of life.

Spinal Muscular Atrophy (SMA)

A hereditary neuromuscular disease known as spinal muscular atrophy (SMA) results in gradual muscle atrophy and weakening due to the spinal cord's loss of motor neurons and specialized nerve cells. SMA may impact a variety of respiratory and movement-related muscles and vary in severity from minor to severe.

Symptoms
- Weakness and atrophy of muscles, particularly in the trunk and limbs
- Hypotonia: insufficient muscular tone
- Trouble getting up, walking, or crawling
- Involuntary muscular contractions or tremors

- Issues with breathing
- Issues with swallowing
- Scoliosis (spinal curvature)

Infants with delayed motor milestones

Causes
- A genetic mutation on chromosome 5 in the survival motor neuron 1 (SMN1) gene

The pattern of autosomal recessive inheritance
- Absence of survival motor neuron (SMN), a protein essential to motor neuron function
- Distinct SMA subtypes (Types I, II, III, and IV) with variable severity according to SMN2 gene copies

Treatments
- Treatments for disease modification, such as onasemnogene abeparvovec-xiii (Zolgensma) and nusinersen (Spinraza)
- Supportive treatment to control symptoms, including respiration and feeding assistance
- Occupational and physical therapy to preserve function and mobility

- Mobility aids and orthoses, among other assistive technology
- Clinical studies looking at genetic methods, gene therapy, and novel medicines
- Multidisciplinary care teams for all-encompassing SMA treatment and support.

Myasthenia Gravis

Myasthenia gravis is an autoimmune disease that causes weariness and muscle weakening. Usually, the affected muscles regulate the movement of the eyes and eyelids, facial expressions, chewing, swallowing, and sometimes breathing. It is brought on by antibodies targeting acetylcholine receptors at the neuromuscular junction, which disrupts the transmission of information between muscles and neurons.

Symptoms
- Weakness in muscles that becomes worse with activity and gets better after rest
- Ptosis (eyelid drooping)

- Diplopia, or seeing twice
- Weakness of the facial muscles
- Trouble swallowing or chewing
- Limb weakness, particularly in the hands and legs
- Weariness and depletion

In extreme situations, dyspnea and respiratory distress

Causes

- Autoimmune disease in which the immune system targets the neuromuscular junction's acetylcholine receptors.
- Thymoma in some individuals or anomalies of the thymus gland
- Genetic susceptibility
- Immune response-triggering environmental variables
- Drugs that interfere with neurotransmission

Treatments

- Acetylcholinesterase inhibitors to raise neuromuscular junction acetylcholine levels

- Medication that suppresses the immune system to alter it
- Thymectomy (surgical removal of the thymus gland).
- Intravenous immunoglobulin treatment or plasmapheresis to eliminate toxic antibodies.
- Supportive treatments, such as speech and physical therapy.
- Constant observation and therapy modification to control symptoms and illness development.

Tourette syndrome

A neurological condition called Tourette syndrome is characterized by tics—repetitive, uncontrollable motions and vocalizations. These tics may be verbal (such as grunting, clearing the throat, or uttering words or phrases) or motor (such as blinking, head jerking, or shoulder shrugging). Their frequency, severity, and complexity can all vary. The onset of Tourette syndrome usually occurs in childhood, and its seriousness might change over time.

Symptoms

- Involuntary motions known as motor tics, which include shoulder shrugging, facial grimacing, and blinking
- Vocal tics, such as throat clearing, grunting, or uncontrollably speaking

- Complex tics such as coprolalia, or inappropriate outbursts, or echolalia, or repeating words
- Tics that fluctuate in severity and frequency over time
- Premonitory cravings or feelings before tics
- Behavioral signs such as attention-deficit/hyperactivity disorder (ADHD) or obsessive-compulsive behaviors
- Stress, exhaustion, or excitement may cause tics to become better or worse.

Causes

- A significant contributing factor to Tourette syndrome is genetics.

- Misfunctions of the neurotransmitter systems, especially those of serotonin and dopamine
- Triggers or environmental variables, such as immunological reactions, infections, or stress during pregnancy.

Disparities in the structure or function of the brain regions responsible for impulses and movement

Treatments
- Behavioral treatment such as exposure response prevention or habit reversal training
- Drugs to treat tics and related symptoms, such as injections of botulinum toxin, alpha-2 adrenergic agonists, or antipsychotics
- In extreme situations, deep brain stimulation
- Supportive treatment for related disorders such as OCD or ADHD
- Assistance and education to help patients and their families deal with the difficulties caused by Tourette syndrome.

Chapter 6

Restless Legs Syndrome

The neurological condition known as restless legs syndrome (RLS) is characterized by an intense need to move the legs and is sometimes accompanied by unpleasant feelings like tingling, crawling, or itching. These symptoms may impair quality of life and interfere with sleep as they often arise or worsen during inactivity or rest, especially in the evening or at night. Leg movement momentarily reduces these feelings.

Symptoms
- Uncomfortable leg sensations, often characterized as itching, crawling, or creeping
- Encourage leg movement to ease pain, which is usually worst at night or when at rest.
- During sleep, restlessness or involuntary leg movements

- Insomnia and sleep disruptions brought on by leg pain
- The intensity of the symptoms varies and might affect everyday activities and quality of life.

Causes
- Primary (idiopathic) RLS, which is connected to hereditary factors but lacks a proven cause
- Secondary RLS linked to ailments such as peripheral neuropathy, iron insufficiency, renal failure, and pregnancy
- A malfunction in the brain's dopamine signaling system, which controls sensation and muscular movement

Treatments
- Changes in lifestyle, such as consistent sleep patterns, abstaining from stimulants, and engaging in regular exercise
- Taking iron supplements if your iron levels are low
- Drugs used to treat symptoms, such as opioids, anticonvulsants, and dopamine agonists

- Try massage, heat or cold treatment, and relaxation methods to reduce pain.
- Cognitive behavioral treatment to enhance sleep hygiene and develop coping mechanisms
- Frequent follow-up visits with a medical professional to discuss therapy modifications depending on symptom response.

Peripheral Neuropathy

Damage to the peripheral nerves, or those not part of the brain and spinal cord, is the hallmark of peripheral neuropathy, a disorder.

Symptoms
- Pain, tingling, or numbness in the hands, feet, or other limbs
- Sensory sensations, such as burning, piercing, or very sensitive to touch
- Loss of coordination or weakening of the muscles
- Lightheadedness or dizziness brought on by

autonomic nerve failure
- Symptoms may be symmetric or asymmetric, affecting one or both sides of the body.

Causes
- Diabetes mellitus is a prevalent cause that results in persistently elevated blood sugar levels, which damages peripheral nerves.
- Alcoholism, exposure to pollutants, and vitamin deficits, particularly with B vitamins
- Immune disorders such as chronic inflammatory demyelinating polyneuropathy (CIDP) and Guillain-Barre syndrome
- Infections such as hepatitis C, Lyme disease, HIV, or shingles
- Nerve compression, recurrent trauma, or other physical trauma

Treatments:
- Dealing with the root cause (e.g., treating dietary deficiencies, managing blood sugar in people with diabetes)
- Painkilling drugs, such as analgesics,

anticonvulsants, and antidepressants
- Occupational therapy and physical therapy to enhance mobility, strength, and coordination
- Nerve blocks or transcutaneous electrical nerve stimulation (TENS) for the treatment of pain
- Modifications to one's way of life, such as consistent exercise, abstaining from alcohol, and eating a balanced diet.

Facial Nerve Palsy (Bell's palsy)

Abdominal palsy, another name for belly palsy, is a disorder marked by weak or paralyzed abdominal muscles. Since the abdominal muscles are essential for maintaining core stability and support, breathing, posture, and movement issues may result.

Symptoms
- Abrupt facial muscular weakness or paralysis, usually on one side of the face
- A sagging corner of the mouth or eyelid
- Having trouble making facial gestures or shutting one eye

- Soreness behind the ears or around the jaw
- Modified taste perception or heightened auditory sensitivity
- Symptoms might appear quickly and peak in a day or two.

Causes.

Although the precise etiology is uncertain, viral infections—specifically the herpes simplex virus (HSV)—are thought to play a factor.
- The function of the face nerve (cranial nerve VII) is disrupted by swelling and inflammation. Pregnancy, diabetes, upper respiratory infections, and a family history of Bell's palsy are risk factors.

Treatments

- Corticosteroids to lessen edema and inflammation around the nerve in the face
- Antiviral drugs if a herpes simplex infection is thought to be present.
- Eye drops and painkillers to control discomfort and prevent dry eyes

- Exercises from physical therapy to maintain muscular tone and avoid contractures
Most instances clear up in a few weeks to months, and there's a strong chance that facial function will be fully restored.

Transverse Myelitis

Transverse myelitis is a neurological condition characterized by spinal cord inflammation, which may cause symptoms including pain, weakness, problems with senses, and bladder dysfunction.

Symptoms
- Abrupt onset of neck or back discomfort
- Modifications in feeling, such as tingling, numbness, or loss in the afflicted region
Paralysis or weakness in the limbs
- Dysfunction of the bowel and bladder
- Trouble balancing or walking
- Frequently happens at a certain level of the spinal cord, resulting in symptoms below that level

Causes
- Autoimmune diseases in which the immune system attacks the spinal cord
- Viral illnesses such as Epstein-Barr virus, varicella-zoster, or herpes
- Bacterial infections, including syphilis or TB
- Reactions after an infection or immunization that cause the spinal cord to become inflamed
Rarely, illnesses like multiple sclerosis that cause demyelinating

Treatments:
- High-dose corticosteroids to inhibit the immune system and lessen inflammation
- Plasma exchange (plasmapheresis), which rids the blood of dangerous antibodies
- Immunomodulatory intravenous immunoglobulin (IVIG) treatment
- Physical treatment to preserve function, strength, and mobility
Treatment of intestinal and bladder problems with drugs or catheterization

- Supportive care for transverse myelitis consequences such as pain and spasticity
- Extended rehabilitation to maximize recovery and standard of living.

Chapter 7

Autoimmune Encephalitis

An uncommon disorder known as autoimmune encephalitis occurs when the body's immune system unintentionally targets healthy brain cells, causing inflammation in the brain and various neurological symptoms.

Symptoms

- Cognitive impairment, memory issues, disorientation, or changed mental state
- Mental health problems such as altered personality, delusions, or hallucinations.

- Abnormal movements, such as dystonia, tremors, or seizures
- Dysautonomia resulting in dysregulation of temperature, blood pressure, or irregular heartbeat
Fever, exhaustion, and headache are possible side effects.

Causes:
- Autoimmune response, in which the immune system unintentionally attacks the brain
- Tumors, other autoimmune illnesses, and viral infections are examples of trigger factors.
- Encephalitis may result from antibodies directed against specific brain proteins.

Treatments
- Immunosuppressive treatments such as plasma exchange, intravenous immunoglobulins, or corticosteroids
- Immunomodulatory medications to control the immune system
- Addressing underlying causes such as tumors or illnesses

- Supportive care for the treatment of symptoms and recovery
- Early identification and treatment are essential for improved results in cases with autoimmune encephalitis.

Creutzfeldt - Jakob disease (CJD)

An uncommon and quickly developing neurodegenerative illness that affects the brain and causes memory loss, cognitive decline, and other neurological symptoms is called Creutzfeldt-Jakob disease.

Symptoms
- Dementia that advances quickly and causes severe disorientation, personality changes, and memory loss

Modifications in behavior, such as agitation, anxiety, or psychosis
- Problems with muscular rigidity, jerky motions, and coordination (myoclonus)
- Distortions in vision, hallucinations, and ultimately blindness

- Problems with speech, weakened muscles, and poor coordination
- Patients may become akinetic and entirely motionless in severe stages.

Causes
- Misfolded proteins, or prion diseases, impact the brain and produce conditions like Creutzfeldt-Jakob disease.
- It may be inherited (associated with mutations in the PRNP gene), spontaneous, or acquired via contact with infected tissues.

The aberrant prion proteins set off a series of actions that result in the degeneration and injury of neurons.

Treatments
- CJD has no known cure; the mainstay of therapy is symptom management.
- To treat anxiety, agitation, or other behavioral issues, doctors may prescribe medication.
- The care goals are to keep the patient

comfortable, control their diet and hydration, and deal with any problems.
- Because the illness progresses quickly, end-of-life care and hospice assistance may be required.

Neurofibromatosis.

A hereditary condition known as neurofibromatosis results in tumors growing on nerves, which may produce a variety of symptoms, including skin, bone, and neurological problems. Neurofibromatosis comes in three varieties: type 1 is the most prevalent, while variants 2 and 3 (also called schwannomatosis) are less frequent.

Symptoms
1. Type 1 neurofibromatosis (NF1):
- Spots of café au lait on the skin
- Numerous benign tumors called neurofibromas on or under the skin
- Cognitive problems and learning difficulties
- Abnormalities of the bones and the spine's curvature

- Gliomas of the optic pathway causing visual issues

2. Type 2 neurofibromatosis (NF2):
- Vestibular schwannomas, or tumors on the nerves responsible for hearing
- Meningiomas, which are tumors on the brain and spinal cord lining.
- Additional malignancies of the brain and spinal cord causing neurological impairments
- Issues with balance and hearing
- Gliomas of the optic pathway causing alterations in vision

Causes
1. NF1:
- Chromosome 17 mutation in the NF1 gene
- Pattern of autosomal dominant inheritance
- Unplanned genetic changes in people without a family background

2. NF2:
- Chromosome 22 mutation in the NF2 gene

- Pattern of autosomal dominant inheritance
Moreover, sporadic mutations may happen.

Treatments
1. NF1:
- Tracking and keeping an eye out for tumor development and consequences
- Treating or removing neurofibromas that are causing symptoms surgically
- Physical treatment for anomalies of the spine and bones
-Genetic guidance about family planning

2. NF2:
- Radiation treatment or surgery for tumors such as vestibular schwannomas
- Cochlear implants or hearing aids for those with hearing loss
- Control of neurological symptoms and balance
- Consistent observation regarding tumor development and consequences
A multidisciplinary strategy involving neurologists, geneticists, oncologists, and other

experts is necessary to effectively care for neurofibromatosis, which addresses the condition's many symptoms and possible consequences.

Rett Syndrome

Girls are affected mainly by the uncommon genetic condition Rett Syndrome, which causes severe neurological and developmental problems. It usually manifests in early infancy, resulting in cognitive and social impairments, respiratory issues, motor difficulties, repetitive hand motions, loss of gained abilities, and other symptoms. Rett syndrome sufferers may need lifetime assistance and care.

Symptoms
Regression is the loss of learned abilities such as motor coordination, social interaction, and intentional hand usage.
- Hand Motions: Common hand motions include washing and wringing.
- Breathing Problems: Unusual breathing

techniques such as apnea or hyperventilation.
- Motor Challenges: Impaired motor function resulting in problems with movement.
Speech Issues: Dysfluency in speech and communication.

Causes
- Genetic Mutation: X chromosome-based mutation in the MECP2 gene.
- X-Linked Dominant Disorder: Because of its inheritance pattern, it primarily affects women.
- Random Mutation: Usually happens seldom, and there is no family history.

Treatments
- Symptomatic Care: Pay close attention to controlling symptoms such as breathing problems and movement issues.
- Physical therapy: Supports the preservation of motor function and muscle tone.
- Speech therapy: Promotes language development and improves communication abilities.

Educational Support: Personalized special education programs.
- Behavioral Therapies: Help with social skill development and managing behavioral issues.

Chapter 8
Spinocerebellar Ataxia.

Spinocerebellar ataxia (SCA) is a class of progressive neurodegenerative genetic illnesses that affect balance, coordination, and motor control. It is characterized by degeneration of the spinal cord and cerebellum, which results in symptoms including muscle weakness, tremors, speech abnormalities, and gait abnormalities. Distinct genetic mutations may produce different forms of SCA, each with a variable pace of onset and development. The goals of treatment are to control symptoms and enhance life quality.

Symptoms
- Ataxia: Unsteadiness and poor coordination. Speech difficulties (dysarthria).
- Nystagmus: Uncontrollably moving eyes. Dysphagia is the inability to swallow.

Causes
- Genetic Mutations: The cerebellum and spinal cord are affected by inherited genetic mutations.
- Trinucleotide Repeat Expansion: The expansion of repetitive DNA sequences impairs nerve cells and areas responsible for motor control.

Treatments
- Symptomatic Management: Occupational therapy and physical therapy are used to treat symptoms.
- Speech therapy: Enhances capacity for communication.
- Hereditary counseling: To help impacted people and their families comprehend the hereditary risk and its consequences.

Friedreich's Ataxia.

An uncommon hereditary condition known as Friedreich's ataxia gradually damages the neurological system, impairing coordination, weakening the muscles, and perhaps causing cardiac issues. It is brought on by a mutation that impacts mitochondrial function in a particular gene. Since there is no cure, treatment controls symptoms and enhances quality of life.

Symptoms
- Ataxia: Disruptions to gait and uncoordinated motions.
- Muscle weakening: Increasing weakening of the muscles, especially the legs.
- Loss of Sensation: The arms and legs feel less. Cardiomyopathy, which results in heart problems, is the cause of cardiac symptoms.
Scoliosis: An irregular curvature of the vertebrae.
- Diabetes: A higher chance of contracting the disease.

Causes
- Genetic Mutation: Mitochondrial function is compromised by the inheritance of a mutant frataxin gene.
- GAA Repeat Expansion: The frataxin gene's GAA repeat expansion results in lower amounts of frataxin.

Treatments
- Physical therapy: Supports the preservation of function and mobility.
Occupational therapy: Assists with day-to-day life tasks.
- Heart Monitoring: Routine heart evaluations are done to treat cardiomyopathy.
- speaking therapy: aids with swallowing and speaking problems.
- Genetic counseling: Offers guidance and assistance in understanding inheritance patterns and family planning.

Autism Spectrum Disorder (ASD).

Difficulties with speech, social interaction, and repetitive activities characterize the complex neurodevelopmental condition of autism. The following are some essential ideas to comprehend ASD fully;

Symptoms
- Challenges with Social Communication: Inability to read social signs, carry on conversations, and convey feelings.
-Restricted, repeating Behaviors: sticking to strict routines, focusing on a particular subject, and performing repeating actions or motions.
- Sensory Sensitivities: Increased or decreased receptivity to touch, taste, smell, or sound.

>Conclusion
- Standardized tests, developmental history, and behavioral observations are used to diagnose autism spectrum disorder (ASD).
- Early childhood is when signs of ASD may be seen, and a diagnosis is usually obtained between

the ages of two and three.

> **Causes**
- Genetic Factors: A higher risk of ASD is linked to specific genetic mutations or variants.
- Environmental Factors: ASD may arise as a result of a mother's sickness, prenatal exposure to certain chemicals, or pregnancy-related problems.
- Brain Differences: Research indicates that the structure and connections of the brain may vary in people with ASD.

>Medication and Supervision:
- Behavioral Therapies: People with ASD may benefit from social skills training, occupational therapy, speech therapy, and applied behavioral analysis (ABA), which can all help them communicate and connect with others better.
- Medication: To control symptoms like anxiety, hostility, or hyperactivity, some people may find relief with medication.
- Early Intervention: For those with ASD, early diagnosis and treatment may improve results.

> Assistance and Materials
Support groups, neighborhood initiatives, and instructional materials can significantly assist people with ASD and their families.
Building an inclusive society requires an appreciation and respect for individual diversity.

> Autism Spectrum Continuum
- Autism Spectrum Disorder (ASD) exhibits moderate to severe symptoms. This variation demonstrates the range of difficulties and abilities faced by people with ASD.
Individual characteristics, difficulties, and unique talents of people with ASD must be considered when assessing and meeting their needs. For those with ASD, early identification, intervention, and continued care may improve their quality of life and general well-being.

It has been suggested that children's brain inflammation may play a role in the development of neurological conditions like autism.

Neuroinflammation, or brain inflammation, may cause abnormalities in brain structure and function, impairing normal neurodevelopment processes and leading to neurodevelopmental disorders.

The immune system is essential for controlling inflammation in the brain. Immune system dysregulation may bring on an inflammatory reaction. Inflammation impacts neural circuit formation, neurotransmitter levels, and disruption of neuronal transmission and is essential for healthy brain function.

Some data indicate that neuroinflammation might be involved in the pathophysiology of autism. Research has shown that people with autism have aberrant immunological responses in addition to higher amounts of inflammatory markers in their brains. Researchers are now looking at a possible connection between inflammation and autism due to these results.

It is essential to remember that there is a

complicated and incomplete understanding of the association between brain inflammation and autism. Although some studies have shown that children with autism have neuroinflammation, additional investigation is required to identify the precise processes via which inflammation may play a role in the disorder's development.

The theory that children's brain inflammation may be the root cause of neurological conditions like autism emphasizes the significance of further investigation into the connection between neuroinflammation and neurodevelopmental disorders, as well as the possible consequences for preventative and therapeutic approaches.

Chapter 9

Meningitis

Meningitis is a dangerous illness marked by inflammation of the meninges, the membranes that coat the brain and spinal cord. Usually, an infection—which might be bacterial, viral, or fungal in origin—is the source of this inflammation.

Meningitis symptoms may vary based on the patient's age and the exact source of the infection. However, frequent symptoms include a high fever, stiff neck, intense headache, light sensitivity, changed mental state, nausea, vomiting, and, in rare situations, a rash. In addition, irritability, inadequate eating, and a protruding fontanelle—a soft region on top of the head—may be present in newborns.

If treatment for bacterial meningitis is delayed, it may have significant consequences and is often more severe than viral meningitis. Neisseria meningitidis, Haemophilus influenzae, and Streptococcus pneumoniae are common causes of bacterial meningitis. Meningitis caused by viruses is generally less severe and goes away independently. Fungal meningitis is less prevalent and often affects those with compromised immune systems.

To treat bacterial meningitis, intravenous antibiotics must be given while the patient is hospitalized. Occasionally, corticosteroids may also be used to reduce inflammation. The symptoms of viral meningitis may usually be controlled with rest, water, and over-the-counter painkillers. Usually, no special treatment is needed. Antifungal drugs may be necessary for the treatment of fungal meningitis.

One way to prevent meningitis is to be vaccinated against certain bacterial strains that might cause it, such as the pneumococcal and meningococcal vaccines. Another is to practice good hygiene, including washing your hands and avoiding close contact with ill people.

If you think you or someone you know may have meningitis, getting medical assistance is critical. Timely care can help avoid dangerous consequences and improve results.

Dementia

Dementia is a gradual neurological disorder that impairs behavior, memory, and cognition. Consequently, a person's capacity to carry out everyday tasks declines. There are several forms of dementia, the most prevalent of which is Alzheimer's disease. There are also frontotemporal dementia, mixed dementia, Lewy body dementia, and vascular dementia.

Dementia symptoms may vary based on the kind and degree of the illness. Still, frequent symptoms include memory loss, trouble speaking and understanding others, confusion, difficulty organizing and planning activities, behavioral and emotional changes, and problems with motor abilities. As dementia worsens, people may find it harder to do daily tasks like eating, dressing, and showering.

There are different causes of dementia, depending on the type. The brain's accumulation of tau tangles and amyloid plaques is a hallmark of Alzheimer's disease. The most common cause of vascular dementia is decreased blood supply to the brain due to diseases such as small vessel disease or stroke. The formation of aberrant protein deposits in the brain is the cause of Lewy body dementia.

The goals of dementia treatment are to control symptoms and enhance quality of life. The majority of dementias presently have no known cure. However, memantine and cholinesterase inhibitors may help control behavioral symptoms and improve cognitive performance. For those with dementia, non-pharmacological therapies, including physical exercise, mental stimulation treatment, and memory therapy, may also be helpful in symptom management and quality of life enhancement. For both the person with dementia and their caretakers, support services like respite care and caregiver support groups may be beneficial.

ND(s) Associated with Preterm Birth.

Delivery before 37 weeks of pregnancy is referred to as preterm birth, and it may result in several neurological issues for the baby. These issues often arise from the baby's nervous system and brain not ultimately maturing before delivery, unlike in a full-term pregnancy. Typical neurological disorders linked to premature birth include;

1. Intraventricular hemorrhage (IVH): Because of the delicate blood arteries in their immature brains, preterm newborns are susceptible to bleeding into the ventricular system of their brains. Lethargy, convulsions, erratic vital signs, and alterations in muscle tone are some of the symptoms of IVH.

2. A brain injury known as periventricular leukomalacia (PVL) damages the white matter around the brain's ventricles. It is often linked to blood vessel injury and inadequate oxygen delivery to the brain in premature newborns. PVL

symptoms might include hearing or visual issues, muscular weakness, and developmental delays.

3. Cerebral palsy: A set of abnormalities affecting posture and mobility, cerebral palsy is more common in preterm newborns. Cerebral palsy may cause tremors, involuntary movements, stiffness or paralysis in the muscles, and impaired coordination.

4. Developmental delays: Babies born before their due date are more likely to delay reaching essential life skills, including walking, talking, and crawling. Early intervention treatments may be necessary to address these delays, which an underdeveloped neurological system may cause. Preterm children may have neurological difficulties due to a variety of factors, including placental anomalies, fetal development limitation, and maternal health disorders, including hypertension or gestational diabetes and infections in the mother or baby. Prematurity also poses a significant risk for neurological issues since it stunts the baby's brain and nervous system development.

To encourage normal development, treatment for neurological problems resulting from preterm delivery focuses on treating the individual symptoms. This might include monitoring the infant's neurological condition, offering speech, occupational, or physical therapy if required, and putting treatments in place to control symptoms like spasms or rigidity in the muscles. In extreme circumstances, specific issues, such as bleeding or hydrocephalus, may need surgical procedures or other medical treatments. For preterm babies at risk of neurological problems, early intervention programs that promote growth and correct deficits may also be helpful.

Neonatal Encephalopathy

A neurological disorder called neonatal encephalopathy affects newborns and is characterized by impaired brain activity. It's a dangerous illness that, if left untreated, may cause long-term issues. A variety of symptoms may be present with neonatal encephalopathy, which is often linked to an underlying etiology that may

call for specific medical interventions. Depending on how severe the illness is, newborn encephalopathy symptoms might vary, but frequent indications could be;
1. Modified state of awareness
2. Seizures or strange motions
3. Inadequate sucking or feeding reaction
4. Either hypertonia (higher muscular tone) or hypotonia (lower muscle tone).
5. Breathing problems
6. Unusual reactions
7. Easily agitated or lethargic
8. Slight jaundice.
9. Overheating or hypothermia.
Neonatal encephalopathy may have a variety of reasons, such as;
1. Hypoxic-ischemic injury: Brain damage may occur when there is insufficient oxygen or blood flow to the brain after birth or in the first few months of life.
2. Infections: Certain viral or bacterial infections and chorioamnionitis may cause maternal infections during pregnancy, raising the risk of

newborn encephalopathy.

3. Metabolic disorders: Neurological difficulties may arise from anomalies in babies' metabolic processes or inborn metabolism errors.

4. Trauma: Encephalopathy may result from head trauma either at birth or in the neonatal period.

5. Hereditary factors: Infants may be more susceptible to neurological problems if they have certain hereditary disorders.

The underlying cause must be addressed to treat newborn encephalopathy, and symptoms must be managed with supportive treatment.

Treatment options vary based on the severity of the illness and may include;

1. Keep an eye on neurological health and vital signs
2. Supporting breathing and preserving oxygen levels
3. Using anticonvulsant medicines to manage seizures
4. Provide hydration and feeding assistance
5. Keeping an eye on and controlling body temperature

6. Taking care of metabolic abnormalities.
7. Deciding whether more diagnostic testing or neuroimaging investigations are necessary
8. Delivering early intervention treatments and developmental support to achieve long-term neurodevelopmental objectives

Babies may need intense care in a neonatal intensive care unit (NICU) for careful observation and specialist treatment in situations of severe newborn encephalopathy. Depending on the severity of the problem, the underlying etiology, and the promptness of management, there are different outcomes for neonatal encephalopathy. Improving results and avoiding long-term neurological problems need early detection and treatment of newborn encephalopathy.

Chapter 10

Four Major Brain Disorders Concerning Neurological Disorders

Numerous variables, including genetic, environmental, lifestyle, and developmental ones, might contribute to brain diseases. The following four leading causes of neurological illnesses involving the brain are as follows:

> Genetic Factors:

- Neurodegenerative Diseases: People who have certain forms of ataxia, Alzheimer's, Parkinson's, or Huntington's disease are more likely to develop neurodegenerative illnesses due to genetic abnormalities.
- Channelopathies: Disorders like migraine and epilepsy may result from genetic defects in ion channels.
- Genetic Syndromes: Disorders with genetic roots that affect brain development include Rett syndrome and Down syndrome.

> Environmental Factors:

- Toxic Exposure: Neurological diseases such as cognitive deficiencies, developmental delays, or neurobehavioral disorders may result from exposure to environmental toxins such as lead, mercury, or pesticides.
- Head Trauma: Concussions, post-concussion syndrome, and chronic traumatic encephalopathy are just a few of the brain illnesses that may arise from traumatic brain injuries (TBIs) sustained in sports-related incidents or accidents.

> **Lifestyle Factors:**

- Diet and Nutrition: Unhealthy eating practices may exacerbate disorders, including neurodegenerative diseases, stroke risk, and cognitive loss.
- Substance Abuse: Abuse of drugs and alcohol may result in mental illnesses, addiction, or cognitive decline.
- Insufficient Exercise: Living a sedentary lifestyle and doing little exercise might raise your chance of developing diseases like depression, stroke, or cognitive loss.

> **Developmental Factors:**

- Prenatal Exposure: During pregnancy, infections, poisons, or illnesses affecting the mother's health might have an impact on the developing fetus's brain, potentially resulting in problems such as intellectual impairments or autism spectrum disorders.
- Early Childhood Events: Neglect, trauma, or adverse events throughout early life may affect brain development and raise the possibility of mental health conditions, including PTSD, anxiety, or depression.
- Neonatal Issues: Learning difficulties, cerebral palsy, and developmental delays may be the outcome of premature delivery, low birth weight, or birth problems. To diagnose, treat, and prevent neurological illnesses via focused therapies, lifestyle changes, genetic counseling, and early intervention techniques, it is essential to comprehend various causes of brain disorders.

How New Neurological Disorder and FRYL Gene Variant are associated.

The protein-coding FRYL (FRYL-like Transcription Coactivator) gene is involved in several biological functions, such as the development and control of gene expression. Neurological problems may result from variations or mutations in the FRYL gene. However, precise correlations may not yet be fully established. This is how a novel neurological condition may be connected to a variation in the FRYL gene:

> Functions of the FRYL Gene:
- The FRYL gene encodes a protein that influences the expression of many genes in the brain and nervous system by participating in gene transcription and co-activation.

> Impact of Variants:
- The FRYL gene is susceptible to variations or mutations that impair its regular expression or function, which may result in aberrant protein interactions or gene regulation in nervous system

cells.

> Neurological Manifestations:

Neurological problems may result from variations in the FRYL gene that affect synapse function, neuronal development, or other brain processes.

> Potential Disorder:

- A novel neurological illness with symptoms including motor dysfunction, cognitive impairment, or sensory abnormalities might be caused by a mutation in the FRYL gene.

> Research and Validation:

- Additional investigation, genetic studies, and functional analysis are necessary to determine the exact processes and consequences of the variation in brain function and establish a definitive connection between a variant of the FRYL gene and a particular neurological condition.

Overall, changes in critical brain pathways caused by gene variations such as FRYL may be linked to neurological illnesses; studying these relationships might shed light on the emergence and management of novel neurological disorders.

Blood-based biomarkers; new outlook for neurological disorders.

Blood is essential for diagnosing and treating neurological illnesses. Developments in blood-based biomarkers are transforming the detection, tracking, and treatment of neurological diseases. The following are some ways blood influences the revised prognosis for neurological disorders.

1. Biomarker discovery: Scientists are finding more and more indicators in blood that correspond to various neurological conditions. These biomarkers help track the development of diseases, determine how healthy treatments are working, and make early diagnoses.

2. Liquid biopsies: Blood samples are a noninvasive method for identifying and tracking neurological conditions. Brain tumors and other neurological disorders may be diagnosed by liquid biopsies, which examine circulating tumor cells, cell-free DNA, and other macromolecules in the blood.

3. Personalized treatment: Blood tests may be used to find genetic mutations or other molecular markers that indicate how a patient will react to certain medications. This individualized strategy makes targeted therapy selection possible, enhancing treatment results and lowering the risk of adverse effects.

4. Drug development: In clinical trials, blood-based biomarkers are also being utilized to evaluate the efficacy of novel medications for neurological illnesses. Drug development may be sped up by using these indicators to assist researchers in choosing individuals who are most likely to benefit from a particular therapy.

5. Disease monitoring Blood tests may provide current details on the course of a disease and how well a medication works. Clinicians may modify treatment strategies to improve patient outcomes by tracking changes in blood biomarkers over time.

Blood-based biomarkers are a potential tool in the new landscape of neurological illnesses, providing noninvasive, economical, and effective diagnosis, monitoring, and treatment. This field of study holds great promise for advancing neurological disease treatment.

Neurocrine Bioscience Therapy

The field of neuroscience, known as neurocrine bioscience therapy or neuropharmacology, focuses on investigating how medications impact the central nervous system and how they could be used to treat neurological conditions. Because neurocrine bioscience therapy targets specific neurotransmitter systems, receptors, and communication pathways in the brain, it is an essential tool in treating various neurological diseases.

The following key points illustrate how neurocrine Bioscience therapy is used to treat neurological disorders:

> **Targeted Treatment:** Drugs targeting specific neurobiological pathways implicated in neurological illnesses are used in neurocrine bioscience treatment. These treatments assist in

relieving symptoms and restoring brain function by specifically altering cellular signaling pathways or neurotransmitter systems.

> **Disease Modification:** Neurocrine Bioscience treatment cannot only treat symptoms of certain neurological conditions, such as Parkinson's disease or epilepsy but also change the underlying pathophysiology or slow down the disease's course. This may assist people with specific diseases in having better long-term results.

> **Personalized Medicine:** Developments in neuropharmacology have paved the way for customized therapeutic strategies that consider each patient's unique genetic makeup, biomarkers, and drug response. Neurocrine Bioscience therapy may be made more effective and safe by customizing treatment plans to meet the unique requirements of individual patients.

> **Combination Therapies:** To provide complete care to patients with neurological illnesses, neurocrine bioscience therapy is often utilized with other therapeutic methods, including

physical therapy, psychotherapy, or surgical procedures. Multimodal methods can potentially enhance treatment results by addressing many parts of the condition.

> **Research and Innovation**:

Neuropharmacology research is still being conducted to find new pharmacological targets, create creative treatments, and enhance existing treatments for neurological diseases. The collaborative efforts of neuroscientists, pharmacologists, and clinicians propel developments in the area, making new therapy choices possible.

Because neurocrine bioscience therapy offers individualized, targeted, disease-modifying therapeutic options that may enhance patient outcomes and quality of life, it is essential to managing neurological illnesses.

Conclusion

Millions of people worldwide suffer from neurological illnesses, which pose a severe threat to global health due to their complicated medical, social, and financial implications. Comprehending the complex interplay of the brain, nervous system, and body is crucial to developing innovative treatments for neurological illnesses in America and worldwide.

Significant strides have been achieved in developing novel medicines and treatments for neurological illnesses domestically and internationally.

The treatment of several illnesses, including multiple sclerosis, epilepsy, Alzheimer's disease, Parkinson's disease, and many more, has been entirely transformed by the introduction of innovative pharmacological agents, such as disease-modifying medications, targeted treatments, and gene therapies. Numerous people with neurological illnesses now live a better quality of life because these developments have also renewed optimism for efficient treatment and disease modification.

In addition, universities, pharmaceutical firms, medical service providers, and government organizations worldwide have joined forces to accelerate the advancement of neurology and neuroscience.

Clinical trials, research investigations, and interdisciplinary approaches have made the discovery of new pharmacological targets, biomarkers, and therapeutic techniques possible, which has the potential to revolutionize the treatment of neurological disorders.
Sustained funding for healthcare infrastructure, education, and research will be crucial to advancing cutting-edge treatments for neurological illnesses domestically and internationally.

We may work towards a future where all people impacted by neurological diseases can access appropriate therapies, enhancing outcomes, quality of life, and general well-being worldwide.

This can be achieved by promoting cooperation, innovation, and inclusion in neurology.